The Inspired keto Diet Cookbook

50 Delicious Recipes To Burn Fat And Boost Your Metabolism

Melody Pope

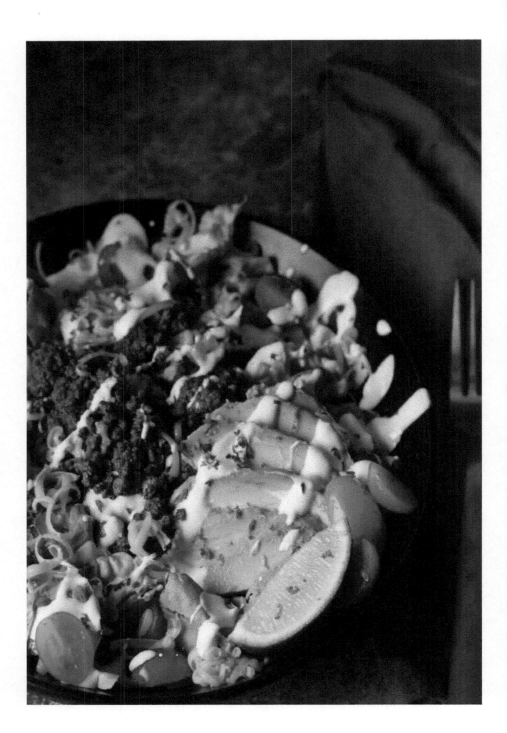

By reading this document, the reader agrees that under no circumstances is the author responsible for any losses, direct or indirect, which are incurred as a result of the use of information contained within this document, including, but not limited to, — errors, omissions, or inaccuracies.

Table of Contents

Mexican Frittata

Preparation time: 10 minutes

Cooking time: 3 hours & 30 minutes

Servings: 6

Ingredients:

- 8 Eggs, large & preferably organic
- ¾ cup Goat Cheese, crumbled
- 4 cups Baby Arugula
- 1/3 cup Milk
- 1 tsp. Oregano, dried
- Sea Salt, as needed
- ½ of 1 Red Onion, medium & sliced thinly
- 1 ¼ cup Roasted Bell Pepper, chopped
- Black Pepper, grounded

Directions:

1. Start by greasing the insides of the slow cooker with butter. After that, crack eggs one by one into a medium-sized mixing bowl. Stir in milk and oregano to the mixing bowl and whisk them gently.

2. Spoon in salt and pepper to it. Stir well. Place the arugula leaves, goat cheese, onion, and roasted bell pepper in the slow cooker. Put the egg batter over the vegetables and spread well. Finally, close the lid and cook for 3 hours on low heat.

Nutrition:

- Calories: 164
- Fat: 12g
- Carbohydrates: 3g
- Protein: 11g

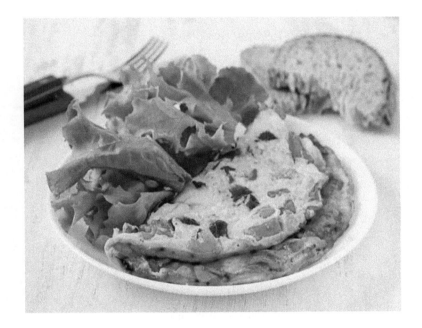

Keto Granola

Preparation time: 10 minutes

Cooking time: 2 hours & 15 minutes

Servings: 12

Ingredients:

- ½ cup Pecans, raw
- 1 tsp. Cinnamon, grounded
- 1/3 cup Coconut Oil
- ½ cup Almonds, raw
- 1 cup Coconut, shredded & unsweetened
- 1 tsp. Vanilla Extract
- 1 cup Sunflower Seeds
- ½ cup Walnuts, raw
- 1 cup Pumpkin Seeds
- ½ cup Hazelnuts, raw
- 1 tsp. Vanilla Stevia
- ½ cup Swerve Sweetener
- ½ tsp. Salt

Directions:

1. To start with, power the crockpot to low heat. Add oil to the crockpot and once it is melted, stir in stevia and vanilla extract. Mix.

2. Then, spoon in all the nuts, shredded coconut, and seeds to the crockpot. Give everything a good stir. Now, sprinkle the cinnamon, salt, and swerve over the nut's seeds mixture.

3. Mix them well and close the lid. Cook within 2 hours on low heat or until the seeds-nut mixture is roasted and browned. Finally, remove it from the crockpot and allow it to cool completely before being stored.

Nutrition:
- Calories: 337
- Fat: 31.6g
- Carbohydrates: 4.8g
- Proteins: 7.9g

Zucchini Bread

Preparation time: 15 minutes

Cooking time: 3 hours

Servings: 10

Ingredients:

- ½ tsp. Vanilla Extract
- 1 1/3 cup Almond Flour
- 2 ½ cup zucchini, finely shredded
- ¼ tsp. Nutmeg
- ½ cup Swerve Sweetener
- ¼ cup Water
- 2 tsp. Baking Powder
- ½ tsp. Salt
- 3 Eggs, large & organic
- ¼ cup Whey Protein Powder, unflavored
- ¼ cup Butter, softened
- 2 tsp. Cinnamon
- ½ tsp. Ginger
- 2/3 cup Coconut, shredded

Directions:

1. For making this bread, place the shredded zucchini in a colander over a bowl. Add salt and mix it well. Allow it to drain for an hour and then squeeze out as much water as possible. Keep it aside.

2. Mix sweetener, nutmeg, almond flour, ginger, coconut, cinnamon, protein powder, and baking powder in a large mixing bowl. Put butter, zucchini, vanilla extract, egg, and water.

3. Combine everything until everything is well incorporated. Now, grease the insert of the crockpot. After that, pour the batter into the crockpot and spread it out. Cook for 3 hours on low heat. Allow it to cool in the crockpot and then serve.

Nutrition:

- Calories: 238
- Fat: 20.22g
- Carbohydrates: 3.62g
- Proteins: 8.95g

Cauliflower Hash Brown Casserole

Preparation time: 15 minutes

Cooking time: 7 hours 30 minutes

Servings: 10

Ingredients:

- 1 Head of Cauliflower, shredded
- 1 Onion, small & diced
- 12 Eggs, large & organic
- 1 lb. Bacon
- 1 tsp. Salt
- 2 cups Cheddar Cheese, shredded
- ½ tsp. Dry Mustard
- Black Pepper, as needed
- ½ cup Milk

Directions:

1. Begin by greasing the crockpot with butter. Combine eggs, pepper, milk, salt, and dry mustard in a large mixing bowl.

2. Arrange a layer of cauliflower on the bottom portion of the crockpot. On to its top, place a third of the onion. Now, spoon in a third of the sausage and cheese.

3. Repeat the layer until all the fixing is used. Once done with layering, spoon in the egg mixture on top. Cook within 7 hours on low heat or until the egg is set.

13

Nutrition:

- Calories: 245
- Fat: 18.76g
- Carbohydrates: 4.01g
- Proteins: 14.98g

Cauliflower Grits

Preparation time: 5 minutes

Cooking time: 3 hours 15 minutes

Servings: 8

Ingredients:

- 6 cups Cauliflower, chopped into florets
- ½ cup Chicken Stock
- ½ tsp. Black Pepper
- 1 tsp. Sea Salt
- 1 cup Cream Cheese

Directions:

1. Process the cauliflower using a food processor until they are finely processed to 'rice' size. Set it aside. Add all the remaining fixing along with the cauliflower rice into the slow cooker and mix them well. Cook them for 3 hours on low heat. Serve it hot.

Nutrition:

- Calories: 161
- Fat: 10.19g
- Carbohydrates: 3.66g
- Proteins: 3.88g

Broccoli Egg Casserole

Preparation time: 10 minutes

Cooking time: 2 hours 45 minutes

Servings : 6 to 8

Ingredients:

- 4 cups Broccoli florets, small
- ¼ cup Parmesan Cheese, coarsely grated
- ½ cup Cottage Cheese washed & dried
- 9 Eggs, large & organic
- ½ tsp. Salt
- 6oz. Swiss Cheese
- Black Pepper, as needed, grounded

Directions:

1. First, boil the broccoli florets in a pot of salt water for 2 minutes. Drain well. After that, place the cottage cheese in a strainer and pour cold water above it until the curd remains. Drain well. Then, lightly whisk the egg in another mixing bowl.

2. Now, grease the insides of the slow cooker with butter. Arrange the broccoli florets onto the bottom of the crockpot.

3. Once done, top it with cottage cheese first and then with Swiss cheese. Finally, layer it with the beaten egg and spread it across.

4. Season it with salt and pepper. Garnish it with parmesan cheese and close the lid. Cook on low heat for 2 ½ to 3 hours or until the egg is set.

Nutrition:

- Calories: 220
- Fat: 15g
- Carbohydrates: 3.64g
- Proteins: 18g

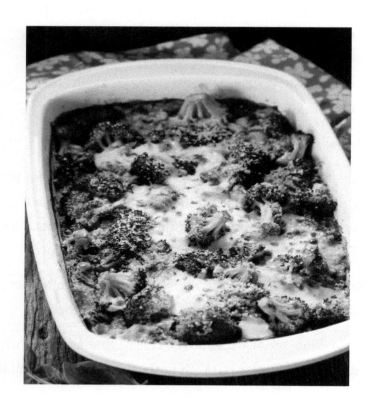

Ham & Egg

Preparation time: 10 minutes

Cooking time: 1 hour 30 minutes

Servings: 4

Ingredients:

- 6 Eggs, large & organic
- ½ cup Heavy Cream
- 1 tbsp. Butter, organic
- 1 cup cheese, shredded
- 1 lb. Ham Steak, trimmed & cubed
- Black Pepper, grounded, as needed
- 2 Green Onion, sliced thinly

Directions:

1. To start with, grease the insides of the slow cooker. Stir in the butter and allow it to melt. After that, add the ham and green onions to a large mixing bowl. Mix well.

2. Then, spoon in the eggs to the bowl and whisk them until combined. Now, pour the heavy cream into this and stir again. Once combined, transfer the egg mixture to the slow cooker.

3. Finally, add salt, pepper, and cheese into this and stir until well incorporated. Cook for 1 hour on high heat. Stir the mixture well and cook for another half an hour until the egg is cooked. Serve hot.

Nutrition:

- Calories: 446
- Fat: 31g
- Carbohydrates: 2.4g
- Proteins: 35g

Pumpkin Pie Bars

Preparation time : 10 minutes

Cooking time: 3 hours 15 minutes

Servings: 16

Ingredients:

To make the crust:

- ½ cup Sunflower Seeds, raw
- 4 tbsp. Butter, organic & softened
- ¾ cup Coconut, shredded & unflavored
- ¼ cup Swerve
- ¼ cup Cocoa Powder, unsweetened
- ¼ tsp. Salt

To make the filling:

- 6 Eggs, large & organic
- 1 tsp. Stevia Extract, pure
- 1 cup Heavy Cream
- 1 tbsp. Pumpkin Pie Spice
- 1 × 29. oz. can of Pumpkin Puree
- 1 tsp. Cinnamon Stevia Extract
- ½ tsp. Salt

Directions:

1. Begin by placing all the ingredients needed to make the crust in a food processor and pulse until it becomes a fine crumble.

2. Then, grease the insides of the crockpot with butter. Spoon in the crust mixture into the crockpot and spread it across.

3. Now, combine all the ingredients needed to make the filling with a mixer in a large bowl. After that, spoon in the filling above the crust.

4. Cook for 3 hours on low heat. Once cooked, allow to cool it in the crockpot for half an hour. Finally, chill them for 2 to 3 hours in the refrigerator. Serve cold.

Nutrition:

- Calories: 151
- Fat: 12.4g
- Carbohydrates: 28g
- Proteins: 5.4g

Coconut Oatmeal

Preparation time: 5 minutes

Cooking time: 8 hours

Servings: 1

Ingredients:

- 1 cup Coconut, shredded & unsweetened
- ½ tsp. Cinnamon
- 2 cups Almond Milk, unsweetened
- ¼ tsp. Liquid Stevia
- ½ tsp. Vanilla Extract
- 2 cups Water
- ¼ cup + 2 tbsp. Coconut Flour

Directions:

1. For making the porridge, you need to combine almond milk, ¼ cup of coconut flour, shredded coconut, cinnamon, and water in the crockpot. Mix well and close the lid.

2. Cook for 8 hours on low heat. Once cooked, stir in the stevia, remaining coconut flour, and vanilla extract to the porridge. Put the bowl in the fridge for some time and then serve.

Nutrition:

- Calories: 113
- Fat: 5g
- Carbohydrates: 3g
- Proteins: 7g

Sour Cream Chicken

Preparation time: 15 minutes

Cooking time: 6 hours

Servings: 4

Ingredients:

- 1 cup of sour cream
- ½ cup of chicken stock
- 1 can of diced green chilis and tomatoes
- 1 batch of taco seasoning
- 2 pounds of chicken breast

Directions:

1. Add all the listed fixing to the slow cooker. Cook on low for 6 hours. Divide onto plates and serve.

Nutrition:

- Calories: 262
- Fat: 13g
- Protein: 32g
- Carbohydrates: 23g

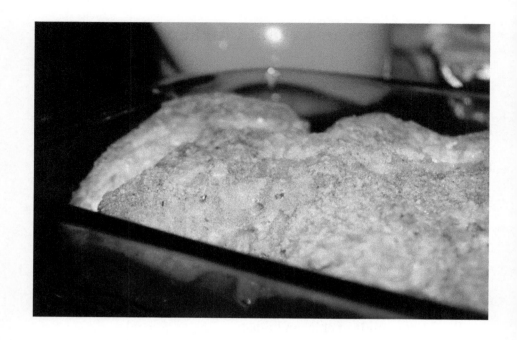

Minced Pork Zucchini Lasagna

Preparation time: 15 minutes

Cooking time: 8 hours

Servings: 4

Ingredients:

- 4 medium zucchinis
- 1 diced small onion
- 1 minced garlic clove
- 2 cups of minced lean ground pork
- 2 cans of Italian diced tomatoes
- 2 tablespoons of olive oil
- 2 cups of shredded Mozzarella cheese
- 1 large egg
- 1 tablespoon of dried basil
- Salt and pepper
- 2 tablespoons of butter

Directions:

1. Slice the zucchini lengthwise into 6 slices. Heat-up the olive oil in a saucepan, and sauté the garlic and onions for 5 minutes. Add the minced meat and cook for a further 5 minutes. Add the tomatoes and cook for a further 5 minutes. Add the seasoning and mix thoroughly.

2. In a small bowl, combine the egg and cheese and whisk. Use the butter to grease the crockpot and then begin to layer the lasagna.

3. The first layer with the zucchini slices, add the meat mixture, and then top with the cheese. Repeat and finish with the cheese. Cover and cook within 8 hours on low.

Nutrition:

- Calories: 398
- Carbohydrates: 10g
- Protein: 23g
- Fat: 30g

Lemon Thyme Chicken

Preparation time: 15 minutes

Cooking time: 4 hours

Servings: 4

Ingredients:

- 10-15 garlic cloves
- 2 sliced lemons
- ½ teaspoon of ground pepper
- 1 teaspoon of thyme
- 3 ½-pound whole chicken

Directions:

1. Arrange the lemon and garlic on the base of a slow cooker. Mix the spices and use them to season the chicken. Put the chicken in the slow cooker. Cover and cook on low within 4 hours. Remove the chicken, let it stand for 15 minutes, and then serve.

Nutrition:

- Calories: 120
- Fat: 8g
- Carbohydrates: 1g
- Protein: 12g

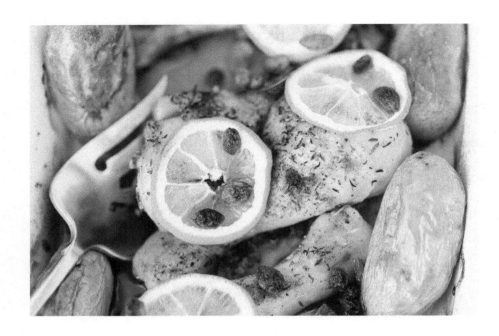

BBQ Ribs

Preparation time : 15 minutes

Cooking time: 8 hours

Servings: 4

Ingredients:

- 3 pounds of pork ribs
- 1 tablespoon of olive oil
- 1 can of tomato paste, 28 ounces
- ½ cup of hot water
- ½ cup of vinegar
- 6 tablespoons of Worcestershire sauce
- 4 tablespoons of dry mustard
- 1 tablespoon of chili powder
- 1 teaspoon of ground cumin
- 1 teaspoon of powdered sweetener of your choice
- Salt and pepper

Directions:

1. Heat the olive oil in a large frying pan and brown the ribs. Place them in the crockpot. In a small bowl, combine the remaining ingredients, whisk thoroughly and pour over the ribs. Cook for 8 hours on low.

Nutrition:

- Calories: 410
- Carbohydrates: 14g
- Protein: 38g
- Fat: 28g

Balsamic Oregano Chicken

Preparation time: 15 minutes

Cooking time: 4 hours

Servings: 6

Ingredients :

- 6 pieces of boneless, skinless chicken
- 2 cans of tomatoes, diced
- 1 large onion, thinly sliced
- 4 garlic cloves
- ½ cup of balsamic vinegar
- 1 tablespoon of olive oil
- 1 tablespoon of dried oregano
- 1 teaspoon of dried rosemary
- 1 teaspoon of dried basil
- ½ teaspoon of thyme
- Salt and pepper

Directions:

1. Mix all the listed fixing except the chicken in a small bowl. Mix them thoroughly. Put the chicken in your slow cooker, then pour the remaining ingredients over the top. Cover and cook on high for 4 hours.

Nutrition:

- Calories: 190
- Fat: 6g
- Carbohydrates: 5g
- Protein: 26g

Bay Leaf Pork Roast Shoulder

Preparation time: 15 minutes

Cooking time: 8 hours

Servings: 4

Ingredients:

- 3 pounds of whole pork shoulder
- 1 can of Italian diced tomatoes
- 1 diced sweet onion
- 3 chopped garlic cloves
- 4 tablespoons of lard
- 1 cup of water
- 1 bay leaf
- ¼ teaspoon of ground cloves
- Salt and pepper

Directions:

1. Place all the above fixing in the crockpot. Cover and cook within 8 hours on low.

Nutrition:

- Calories: 421
- Carbohydrates: 10g
- Protein: 33 g
- Fat: 30g

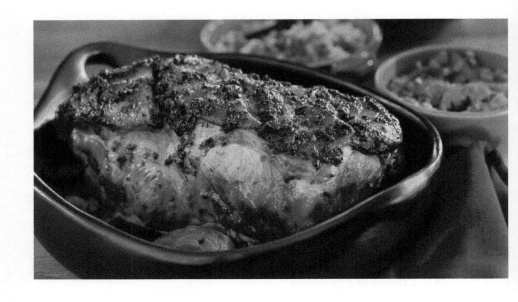

Chicken Breast with Artichoke Stuffing

Preparation time : 15 minutes

Cooking time: 4 hours

Servings: 4

Ingredients:

- 4 boneless, skinless chicken breasts
- 3 cups of finely chopped spinach
- ½ cup of chopped roasted red peppers
- ¼ cup of sliced black olives
- 1 cup of chopped canned artichoke hearts
- 4 ounces of reduced-fat feta cheese
- 1 teaspoon of dried oregano
- 1 teaspoon of garlic powder
- 1 ½ cups of low-sodium chicken broth
- Salt and pepper

Directions:

1. Create a deep slice in the chicken's core or center and season it with salt and pepper. In a small bowl, combine the garlic, feta, oregano, peppers, spinach, and artichoke hearts.

2. Stuff the artichoke mixture into the cut in the chicken and put it into the slow cooker. Cover and cook on low within 4 hours.

Nutrition:

- Calories: 222
- Fat: 7g
- Carbohydrates: 4g
- Protein: 52g

Coconut Turmeric Pork Curry

Preparation time : 15 minutes

Cooking time: 8 hours

Servings: 4

Ingredients:

- 2.2 pounds of cubed pork shoulder
- 1 tablespoon of coconut oil
- 1 tablespoon of olive oil
- 1 diced yellow onion
- 2 minced garlic cloves
- 2 tablespoons of tomato paste
- 1 can of coconut milk, 12 ounces
- 1 cup of water
- ½ cup of white wine
- 1 teaspoon of turmeric
- 1 teaspoon of ginger powder
- 1 teaspoon of curry powder
- ½ teaspoon of paprika
- Salt and pepper

Directions:

1. Heat-up 1 tablespoon of olive oil in a saucepan and sauté the garlic and onions for 3 minutes. Add the pork and brown it, and then add the tomato paste.

2. Mix the remaining ingredients in the crockpot and then add the pork. Cover and cook within 8 hours on low. Divide onto plates and serve

Nutrition:

- Calories: 425
- Carbohydrates: 7g
- Protein: 30g
- Fat: 31g

Pork Chops with Cumin Butter and Garlic

Preparation time: 15 minutes

Cooking time: 4 hours

Servings: 4

Ingredients:

- 3.5 pounds of pork sirloin chops with the bone
- ½ cup of salsa
- 3 tablespoons of butter
- 5 tablespoons of lime juice
- ½ teaspoon of ground cumin
- ¾ teaspoon of garlic powder
- ¾ teaspoon of salt
- ¾ teaspoon of black pepper

Directions:

1. Combine the spices and season the pork chops. Melt the butter in a saucepan and brown the pork chops for 3 minutes on each side.

2. Place the chops into the slow cooker and pour the salsa over the top. Cover and cook on high for 3-4 hours. Divide onto plates and serve.

Nutrition:

- Calories: 364
- Fat: 17g
- Carbohydrates: 3g
- Protein: 51g

Delightful Turkey Basil Meatballs

Preparation time: 15 minutes

Cooking time: 5 hours

Servings: 4

Ingredients:

- 1 package of frozen turkey meatballs
- ½ a cup of bottled yellow and red sweet peppers, chopped and drained
- 1/8 teaspoon of crushed red peppers
- 1 cup of reduced-sodium pasta sauce
- Snipped fresh basil for garnish

Directions:

1. Place all of the ingredients except the basil into the slow cooker. Cover and cook on low for 4-5 hours. Divide onto plates, garnish with the basil and serve.

Nutrition:

- Calories: 68
- Fat: 4g
- Carbohydrates: 3g
- Protein: 6g

Chicken Cooked with Beer

Preparation time: 15 minutes

Cooking time: 8 hours

Servings: 4

Ingredients :

- 1 ½ pound of skinless, boneless chicken breasts
- 1 can of light beer, 12 ounces
- ½ teaspoon of salt
- ½ teaspoon of black pepper
- ½ teaspoon of red pepper flakes
- ½ tablespoon of dried oregano

Directions:

1. Using the oregano, salt, black pepper, and red pepper flakes, season the chicken and arrange it inside the slow cooker. Pour the beer onto the chicken. Cover and cook on low within 6-8 hours. Use two forks to shred the chicken, divide onto plates, and serve.

Nutrition:

- Calories: 139
- Fat: 3g
- Carbohydrates: 0g
- Protein: 28g

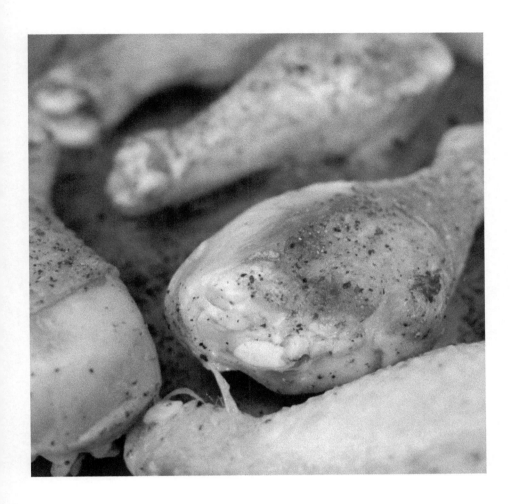

Italian Black Olive Chicken

Preparation time: 15 minutes

Cooking time : 6 hours

Servings: 4

Ingredients:

- 2 pounds of skinless, boneless chicken breasts
- 1 teaspoon of Italian seasoning
- Salt and pepper
- ½ teaspoon of basil
- ¼ teaspoon of red pepper flakes
- 35 pieces of turkey pepperoni, cut in half
- ½ cup of reduced-sodium black olives

Directions:

1. Use the salt and pepper to season the chicken and arrange it in the slow cooker. Add the pepperoni and the olives.

2. Whisk the remaining ingredients and pour on top of the chicken. Cover and cook on low for 6 hours. Shred the chicken, divide onto plates and serve.

Nutrition:

- Calories: 307
- Fat: 10g
- Carbohydrates: 4g
- Protein: 52g

One-Pot Special Meal

Preparation time: 15 minutes

Cooking time: 5 hours

Servings: 4

Ingredients:

- 1 chopped green bell pepper
- 1 cup of fresh spinach
- 1 diced red onion
- 2 minced garlic cloves
- 1 can of Italian tomatoes, diced
- 2 cups of chicken broth
- 2 tablespoons of tomato paste
- 1 cup of sliced black olives
- 1 cup of dry white wine
- 2 bay leaves
- 1 teaspoon of dry basil
- ¼ teaspoon of crushed fennel seeds
- 1 ¾ cups of peeled shrimp, medium size
- 1 ¾ cups of cod, cubed
- Salt and pepper

Directions:

1. Add all of the ingredients except the cod and the shrimp to the crockpot. Cover and cook for 4.5 hours on low. Add the cod and the shrimp, cover, and cook for a further 30 minutes.

Nutrition:

- Calories: 436
- Carbohydrates: 9g
- Protein: 36g
- Fat: 25g

Cinnamon, Coriander, Broccoli Oxtail Pot

Preparation time: 15 minutes

Cooking time: 10 hours

Servings : 4

Ingredients:

- 3 pounds of oxtail cut into small chunks
- 2 tablespoons of olive oil
- 1 diced red onion
- 3 minced garlic cloves
- A piece of ginger, sliced thinly
- 1 can of diced Italian tomatoes
- 1 teaspoon of ground cardamom
- 1 teaspoon of ground cumin
- 1 teaspoon of ground coriander seeds
- ½ teaspoon of cinnamon
- 1 ½ teaspoon of salt
- 1 teaspoon of fresh ground pepper
- 1 cup of hot water and 1 cup of beef broth
- 5 cubed small turnips
- 1 chopped head of broccoli
- 1 cup of diced mushrooms

Directions:

1. Preheat the slow cooker on low. Heat-up the olive oil in a pan, brown the oxtail, and add it to the crockpot. Sauté the onions in the same pan for 5 minutes.

2. When they become translucent, add the ginger and the garlic, cook for a further 1 minute. Once cooked, pour these over the oxtail.

3. Add the rest of the fixing to the saucepan and allow them to boil. Pour the sauce into the slow cooker and stir; the liquid should cover the oxtail. Cover and cook within 8-10 hours on low.

Nutrition:

- Calories: 510
- Carbohydrates: 14g
- Protein: 68g
- Fat: 31g

Ham and Cauliflower Stew

Preparation time: 15 minutes

Cooking time: 4 hours

Servings: 4

Ingredients:

- 3 cups of diced ham
- 16 ounces of frozen cauliflower florets
- ¼ cup of heavy cream
- 14.5 ounces of chicken broth
- ¼ teaspoon of salt
- 4 garlic cloves
- 8 ounces of grated cheddar cheese
- ½ teaspoon of garlic powder
- ½ teaspoon of onion powder
- A dash of pepper

Directions:

1. Place all the above-listed fixing into the slow cooker. Cook on high for 4 hours. Serve.

Nutrition:

- Calories: 320
- Fat: 20.6g
- Carbohydrates: 7.5g
- Fiber: 3g
- Protein: 23.3g

Yogurt Turkey Meatballs

Preparation time: 15 minutes

Cooking time: 7 hours

Servings : 6

Ingredients:

For the meatballs:

- 1¼ pounds ground turkey
- 1 cup crumbled feta cheese
- ½ cup finely chopped walnuts
- ½ cup minced fresh mint
- ¼ cup grated onion
- 4 garlic cloves, minced
- 3 tablespoons paprika
- 1 tablespoon ground cumin
- 1½ teaspoons kosher salt
- 1 teaspoon freshly ground black pepper
- ¼ to ½ teaspoon cayenne pepper
- 2 tablespoons extra-virgin olive oil
- 1 onion, halved and thinly sliced
- 1 cup chicken broth

For the sauce:

- 1 cup plain full-fat Greek yogurt
- 2 tablespoons tahini

- 1 tablespoon freshly squeezed lemon juice
- ½ teaspoon kosher salt
- 1 tablespoon extra-virgin olive oil 1 teaspoon za'atar (optional)
- ½ teaspoon ground sumac (optional)

Directions:

1. In a large bowl, stir the ground turkey, feta, walnuts, mint, onion, garlic, paprika, cumin, salt, black pepper, and cayenne pepper. Form the mixture into about 24 oblong meatballs.

2. In the slow cooker insert, combine the olive oil and onion and spread to cover the cooker's bottom. Top with the meatballs. Pour in the chicken broth. Cover and cook within 7 hours on low.

3. Mix the yogurt, tahini, lemon juice, and salt in a small bowl. Garnish the sauce with a drizzle of olive oil and a sprinkling of za'atar and sumac (if using). Serve the meatballs hot, with the sauce alongside for dipping.

Nutrition:

- Calories: 443
- Fat: 35g
- Carbs: 9g
- Protein: 25g

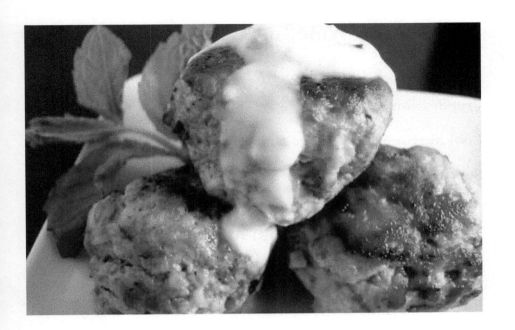

Parsley Wine Tomato-Braised Tuna

Preparation time: 15 minutes

Cooking time: 2 hours & 30 minutes

Servings: 8

Ingredients:

- 2 tuna fillets (3 pounds)
- ½ cup olive oil
- 1 small red onion, chopped
- 6 garlic cloves, minced
- 3 cups gluten-free, sugar-free tomato sauce
- 1 cup dry white wine
- 6 tablespoons drained and rinsed capers
- 4 tablespoons chopped fresh parsley
- 2 bay leaves
- Sea salt
- Freshly ground black pepper

Directions:

1. Place the tuna in a bowl of cold salted water to soak for about 12 minutes. Drain well and pat dry using paper towels.

2. Place a skillet over a medium-high flame and heat 2 tablespoons of oil. Sauté the onion and garlic until the onion is translucent. Transfer into the slow cooker.

3. Stir the wine, tomato, marinara sauce, capers, bay leaves, and parsley into the slow cooker. Cover and cook within 1 hour on high.

4. Put the skillet over medium-high heat and heat the rest of the oil. Brown the tuna fillets all over, then place into the slow cooker. Cover and cook for 1 hour and 30 minutes on high, or until the tuna is cooked.

Nutrition:

- Calories: 155
- Fat: 16.5g
- Carbs: 8g
- Protein: 40g

Garlic Cabbage Beef Soup

Preparation time : 15 minutes

Cooking time : 10 hours

Servings: 6

Ingredients:

- 2 tablespoons coconut oil
- 8 ounces beef stew meat, diced
- Kosher salt
- Freshly ground black pepper
- 8 ounces smoked beef sausage, diced
- 1 onion, finely chopped
- 3 cups shredded cabbage
- 2 cups beef broth
- 1 (15-ounce) can tomato sauce
- 2 garlic cloves, minced
- 2 bay leaves
- 3 tablespoons chopped fresh parsley
- 1 cup sour cream

Directions:

1. Warm-up coconut oil over medium-high heat in a large skillet. Generously season the meat with salt and pepper and add it to the skillet, along with the sausage.

2. Cook until the meat is browned on all sides, about 6 minutes. Transfer the beef and sausage to the slow cooker.

3. Move it back to the skillet to medium-high heat and add the onion. Sauté until softened, about 4 minutes. Transfer the onion to the slow cooker.

4. Add the cabbage, beef broth, tomato sauce, garlic, and bay leaves to the slow cooker. Cover and cook for 8 to 10 hours on low. Discard the bay leaves and serve hot, garnished with the parsley and a dollop of sour cream.

Nutrition:

- Calories: 329
- Fat: 26g
- Carbs: 9g
- Protein: 16g

Mushrooms & Bell Pepper Cheesesteak

Preparation time : 15 minutes

Cooking time: 8 hours

Servings: 6

Ingredients:

- 2 tablespoons coconut oil
- 1 onion, thinly sliced
- 8 ounces cremini or button mushrooms, sliced
- 1 green bell pepper, strips
- 1 red bell pepper, strips
- 1½ pounds rib-eye steak
- ¾ teaspoon kosher salt
- ¾ teaspoon freshly ground black pepper

Directions:

1. In a large skillet, warm up the coconut oil over medium-high heat. Sauté the onion until beginning to soften, about 3 minutes.

2. Put the mushrooms, then continue to sauté until the mushrooms begin to brown, about 5 minutes. Transfer the mixture to the slow cooker.

3. Put the green plus red bell peppers in the slow cooker and stir to mix. Return the skillet to medium-high heat. Flavor the steak with the salt and pepper and add it to the skillet.

4. Cook until browned, within 2 minutes per side. Transfer the steak to the slow cooker, placing it on top of the vegetables. Cover and cook within 8 hours on low.

5. Remove the steak from the cooker and let it rest for a couple of minutes. Leave the slow cooker on and keep it covered.

6. Slice the steak into thin strips and return them to the slow cooker. Place the provolone cheese over the top, replace the cover, and let it sit for a few minutes until the cheese is melty. Serve hot.

Nutrition:
- Calories: 734
- Fat: 59g
- Carbs: 8g
- Protein: 43g

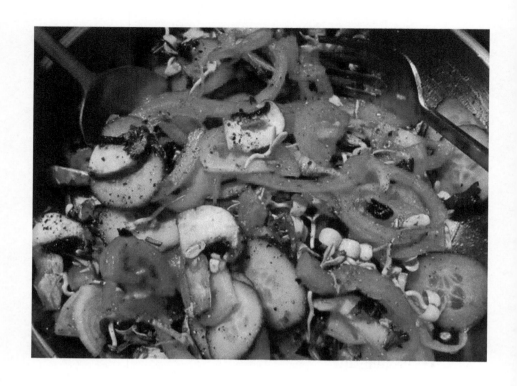

Lemon Garlic Shrimp Scampi

Preparation time: 15 minutes

Cooking time: 1 hour & 30 minutes

Servings: 6

Ingredients:

- 1 lb. raw shrimp, peeled and deveined
- Juice of one fresh lemon
- 1/2 cup chicken broth
- 3 minced garlic cloves
- 4 tbsp butter
- 2 tbsp fresh parsley
- Salt and pepper as desired

Directions:

1. Adjust the heat of the slow cooker to high. Combine the chicken broth, lemon juice, butter, garlic, parsley, salt, and pepper in the crockpot. Stir thoroughly. Put the shrimp in, mixing well. Cook within 1 hour and 30 minutes. Serve.

Nutrition:

- Calories: 250
- Fat: 13.7g
- Carb: 4.6g
- Protein: 27g

Curry Beef

Preparation time: 15 minutes

Cooking time: 8 hours

Servings: 6

Ingredients:

- 1 cup diced tomatoes
- 1 (14-ounce) can coconut milk
- 1/3 cup water
- ¼ cup coconut oil, melted
- ¼ cup tomato paste
- 1 onion, diced
- 6 garlic cloves, minced
- 3 tablespoons grated fresh ginger
- 2 tablespoons ground cumin
- 1 teaspoon paprika
- 1 teaspoon kosher salt
- ½ teaspoon ground turmeric
- ½ teaspoon ground cardamom
- ½ teaspoon ground cinnamon
- ½ teaspoon ground cloves
- ½ teaspoon cayenne pepper
- ¼ teaspoon ground nutmeg
- 1 (1½-pound) beef chuck roast, cut into ½-by-2-inch strips
- 1/3 cup chopped fresh cilantro

Directions:

1. In the slow cooker, stir the tomatoes, coconut milk, water, coconut oil, and tomato paste. Add the onion, garlic, ginger, cumin, paprika, salt, turmeric, cardamom, cinnamon, cloves, cayenne, and nutmeg.

2. Add the beef and toss to mix well. Cover and cook within 8 hours on low. Serve hot, garnished with the cilantro.

Nutrition:

- Calories: 547
- Fat: 46g
- Carbs: 12g
- Protein: 26g

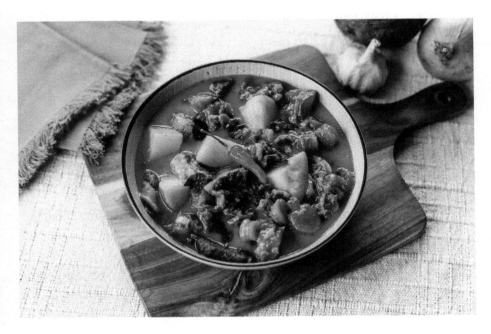

Heavy Creamy Herb Pork Chops

Preparation time: 15 minutes

Cooking time: 8 hours

Servings: 4

Ingredients:

- ¾ cup chicken or beef broth
- 2 tablespoons coconut oil, melted
- 1 tablespoon Dijon mustard
- 2 garlic cloves, minced
- 1 tablespoon paprika
- 1 tablespoon onion powder
- 1 teaspoon dried oregano
- 1 teaspoon dried basil
- 1 teaspoon dried parsley
- 1 onion, thinly sliced
- 4 thick-cut boneless pork chops
- 1 cup heavy (whipping) cream

Directions:

1. In the slow cooker, stir the broth, coconut oil, mustard, garlic, paprika, onion powder, oregano, basil, and parsley.

2. Add the onion and pork chops and toss to coat. Cover and cook within 8 hours on low or 4 hours on high. Transfer the chops to a serving platter.

3. Transfer the remaining juices and onion in the slow cooker to a blender, add the heavy cream, and process until smooth. Put the sauce over the pork chops, then serve hot.

Nutrition:
- Calories: 470
- Fat: 32g
- Carbs: 7g
- Protein: 39g

Mushroom Beef Stroganoff

Preparation time: 15 minutes

Cooking time: 8 hours

Servings : 6

Ingredients:

- 2 pounds beef stew meat, cut into 1-inch cubes
- 4 bacon slices, diced
- 8 ounces cremini or button mushrooms, quartered
- 1 onion, halved and sliced
- 2 garlic cloves, minced
- 1 cup beef broth
- ¼ cup tomato paste
- 1 teaspoon smoked paprika
- ½ teaspoon kosher salt
- ¼ teaspoon freshly ground black pepper
- 1½ cups sour cream
- 2 tablespoons minced fresh parsley

Directions:

1. In the slow cooker, stir the beef, bacon, mushrooms, onion, garlic, beef broth, tomato paste, paprika, salt, and pepper. Cover and cook within 8 hours on low. Stir in the sour cream, then serve hot, garnished with the parsley.

Nutrition:

- Calories: 594
- Fat: 47g
- Carb: 7g
- Protein: 35g

Ginger Cream Sauce Pork Loin

Preparation time: 15 minutes

Cooking time: 8 hours

Servings: 6

Ingredients:

For the pork:

- 1 tablespoon erythritol
- 2 teaspoons kosher salt
- 1 teaspoon garlic powder
- 1 teaspoon ground ginger
- ½ teaspoon ground cinnamon
- ½ teaspoon ground cloves
- ½ teaspoon red pepper flakes
- ¼ teaspoon freshly ground black pepper
- 1 (2-pound) pork shoulder roast
- ½ cup of water

For the sauce:

- 2 tablespoons unsalted butter
- 3 tablespoons minced fresh ginger
- 2 shallots, minced
- 1 tablespoon minced garlic
- 2/3 cup dry white wine
- 1 cup heavy (whipping) cream

69

Directions:

1. In a small bowl, stir the erythritol, salt, garlic powder, ginger, cinnamon, cloves, red pepper flakes, and black pepper. Rub the seasoning mixture all over the pork and place it in the slow cooker.

2. Pour the water into the cooker around the pork. Cover and cook within 8 hours on low. Remove, then let it rest for about 5 minutes.

3. While the pork rests, melt the butter in a small saucepan over medium heat. Stir in the ginger, shallots, and garlic.

4. Add the white wine and bring to a boil. Cook, stirring, until the liquid is reduced to about ¼ cup, about 5 minutes.

5. Mix in the heavy cream, then continue to boil, stirring until the sauce thickens, 3 to 5 minutes more. Slice the pork and serve it with the sauce spooned over the top.

Nutrition:

- Calories: 488
- Fat: 40g
- Carb: 5g
- Protein: 27g

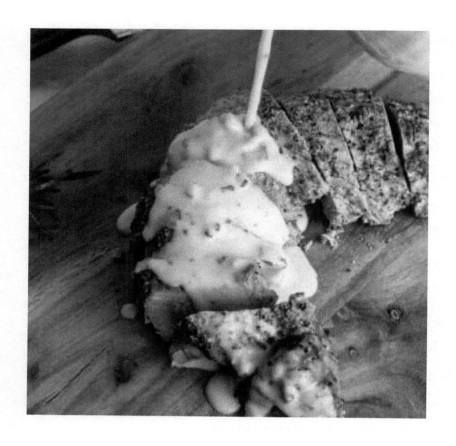

Toasted Almond Braised Beef

Preparation time: 15 minutes

Cooking time: 9 hours

Servings: 6

Ingredients:

- ¼ cup of coconut oil
- 1 medium onion, diced
- 2 teaspoons ground cumin
- 1½ teaspoons kosher salt
- ½ teaspoon freshly ground black pepper
- ½ teaspoon ground cinnamon
- ½ teaspoon ground ginger
- 1 cup dry red wine
- 1 (1¼-pound) beef chuck roast, cut into 2-inch pieces
- Grated zest and juice of 1 orange
- 1 cup heavy (whipping) cream
- 5 tablespoons unsalted butter
- ½ cup ground toasted almonds
- ¼ cup chopped fresh cilantro

Directions:

1. In a large skillet, warm-up coconut oil over medium-high heat. Add the onion and sauté until soft, about 5 minutes. Add the cumin, salt, pepper, cinnamon, and ginger. Sauté for 1 minute more.

2. Mix in the red wine, then boil within 1 to 2 minutes, scraping up any browned bits from the pan's bottom. Transfer the mixture to the slow cooker.

3. Stir in the beef, orange zest, and orange juice. Cover and cook for 9 hours on low or 4½ hours on high.

4. Stir in the heavy cream plus butter until the butter melts, and both are well incorporated. Serve hot, garnished with the almonds and cilantro.

Nutrition:

- Calories: 747
- Fat: 56g
- Carbs: 9g
- Protein: 47g

Coconut Pumpkin Pork Stew

Preparation time: 15 minutes

Cooking time: 8 hours

Servings: 8

Ingredients:

- 2 tablespoons coconut oil
- 1½ pounds boneless pork ribs
- Kosher salt
- Freshly ground black pepper
- ½ onion, chopped
- 1 garlic clove, minced
- 1 jalapeño pepper, seeded and minced
- 1 teaspoon minced fresh ginger
- 1½ cups chicken broth
- 3 cups canned coconut milk
- 1 cup pumpkin purée
- ¼ cup all-natural peanut butter
- ¼ cup erythritol
- 1 teaspoon freshly squeezed lime juice
- ¼ cup chopped fresh cilantro
- ½ cup chopped toasted peanuts

Directions:

1. In a large skillet, heat-up coconut oil over medium-high heat. Flavor the pork with salt and pepper and add it to the skillet. Cook until browned on both sides, about 6 minutes. Transfer to the slow cooker.

2. Return the skillet to medium-high heat and add the onion, garlic, jalapeño, and ginger. Sauté until the onions are softened, about 3 minutes. Mix in the chicken broth and boil within 1 minute.

3. Stir in the coconut milk, pumpkin, peanut butter, and erythritol until smooth. Pour the mixture into the slow cooker. Cover and cook for 8 hours on low.

4. Remove the meat from the slow cooker, cut it into bite-size pieces, or shred it using two forks. Return the meat to the cooker. Stir in the lime juice. Serve hot, garnished with the cilantro and peanuts.

Nutrition:

- Calories: 492
- Fat: 41g
- Carb: 11g
- Protein: 24g

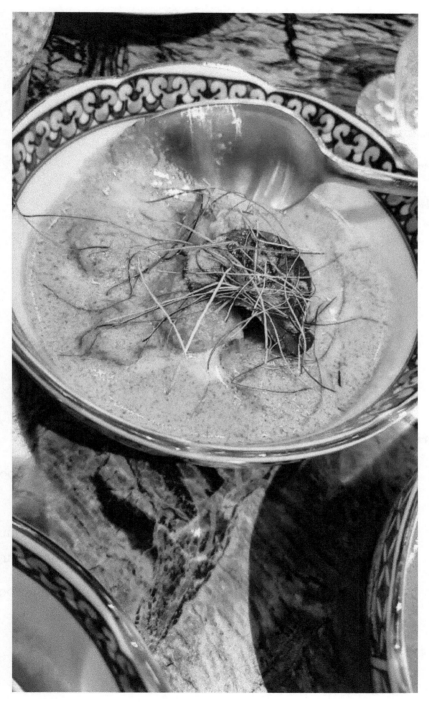

Ginger Spinach Chicken

Preparation time: 15 minutes

Cooking time: 5 hours

Servings: 8

Ingredients:

- 1/2 cup liquid aminos
- 1 tbsp fresh ginger, minced
- 8 chicken thighs
- 2 cups of water
- 1 tbsp garlic powder
- 1 tsp blackstrap molasses
- Salt and pepper to taste
- 2 cups spinach, whole leaves

Directions:

1. Mix the water and liquid aminos. Put this mixture in the crockpot. Add all the other spices and mix this in thoroughly as well.

2. Place the chicken thighs in the liquid in the slow cooker. Adjust the heat setting to high heat and put the lid on. Cook for 5 hours.

3. Add the spinach to the mixture in the crockpot. Recover and cook on high for ten minutes, stirring occasionally. Serve hot.

Nutrition:

- Calories: 472
- Fat: 35.7g
- Carb:3.8g
- Protein: 32.7g

Ghee Salmon with Fresh Cucumber Salad

Preparation time: 15 minutes

Cooking time: 3 hours

Servings: 8

Ingredients:

- 4 x 4oz Wild salmon fillets
- 2 tsp Tandoori spice
- 1 tsp salt
- 1 tsp black pepper
- 4 tbsp ghee
- Cucumber Salad
- 1 English cucumber
- 1 cup arugula
- ½ cup parsley
- ¼ cup lemon juice
- 2 tbsp extra virgin olive oil

Directions:

1. Heat-up ghee in a skillet over medium heat along with tandoori spice for a minute. Place salmon fillets in the slow cooker, skin side down, sprinkle with salt, black pepper, and pour Tandoori butter over salmon.

2. Cook on high for 3.5 hours. While salmon is cooking, dice the cucumber, and toss with arugula, parsley, lemon juice, and extra virgin olive oil. Serve salmon with fresh cucumber salad.

Nutrition:

- Calories: 413
- Carbs: 4g
- Fat: 34g
- Protein: 25g

Short Ribs

Preparation time: 15 minutes

Cooking time: 4 hours

Servings: 8

Ingredients:

- 4lbs. short ribs, bone-in
- 8 peppercorns
- 2 cups low-sodium beef
- 1 onion, diced
- 2 carrots, peeled, diced
- 2 celery stalks, diced
- 4 cloves, minced
- 1 tsp thyme
- 1 tsp rosemary
- 2 bay leaves
- 2 tsp salt
- 2 tsp black pepper
- Extra virgin olive oil

Directions:

1. Heat-up 4 tbsp extra virgin olive oil in a skillet. Add onions and garlic, and sauté until brown. Place onion mixture in the slow cooker, add short ribs, carrots, celery stalk, cloves, thyme, rosemary, peppercorns, bay leaves, salt, and black pepper. Cook on high for 4 hours.

Nutrition:
- Calories: 520
- Fat: 24g
- Carbs: 3.7g
- Protein: 67g

Cilantro Chili Verde

Preparation time: 15 minutes

Cooking time: 7 hours

Servings: 8

Ingredients:

- 1½lbs. pork shoulder
- ½ lb. sirloin, cubed
- 4 Anaheim chilis, stemmed
- 6 minced garlic cloves
- ½ cup cilantro, chopped
- 2 onions, peeled and sliced
- 2 tomatoes, chopped.
- 1 tbsp tomato paste
- 1 lime
- 1 tbsp cumin
- 1 tbsp oregano
- Extra virgin olive oil

Directions:

1. Slice pork shoulder into 1" cubes, and set slow cooker to medium. Heat-up four tbsp extra virgin olive oil in a skillet, add onions, Anaheim chilies, garlic, and sauté for 2 minutes.

2. Place skillet mixture into the slow cooker, add pork shoulder, sirloin, and stir. Add tomatoes, cilantro, tomato paste, cumin, oregano, and salt to the pot. Cover and cook for 7 hours. Squeeze a little lime in each bowl when serving.

Nutrition:

- Calories: 262
- Fat: 16g
- Carbs: 6g
- Protein: 23g

Thai Zucchini Lasagna

Preparation Time: 45 minutes

Cooking Time: 4 hours

Servings: 8

Ingredients:

For the zoodles:

- 4 large zucchinis
- 1 tbsp salt

For the lasagna:

- 2 tbsp coconut oil
- 1-pound extra-lean ground turkey
- 1 cup onion, diced
- 1 tbsp + 2 tsp fresh garlic, minced
- 1/2 tbsp fresh ginger, minced
- Pepper
- 1 cup light coconut milk
- 1/4 cup natural creamy peanut butter
- 1/4 cup reduced-sodium soy sauce
- 2 tbsp coconut sugar
- 1 tbsp rice vinegar
- 1 tbsp fresh lime juice
- 1 tbsp fish sauce
- 1-2 tbsp sriracha
- 15oz. light ricotta cheese

- 1 large egg
- 1/2 cup cilantro, roughly chopped
- 2 cups Nappa cabbage, roughly chopped
- 1/2 cup water chestnuts, diced
- 8 ounces mozzarella cheese, grated
- 1 large red pepper, diced

For garnish:

- Cilantro, diced
- Green onion, diced
- Roasted peanuts, diced
- Bean sprouts, roughly chopped

Directions:

1. Warm-up oven to 350 degrees. Cut the zucchini into thin using a mandolin, about 1/8 inch thick. Lay them out flat onto cookie sheets and sprinkle with 1 tbsp salt.

2. Bake within 15-20 minutes. Warm-up coconut oil over medium-high heat in the large pan. Put in the ground turkey, onion, garlic, ginger, plus a pinch of pepper. Cook within 10-12 minutes.

3. Once cooked, put the coconut milk, peanut butter, soy sauce, coconut sugar, rice vinegar, lime juice, fish sauce, plus 1 tbsp of the sriracha. Boil within 3 minutes. Adjust the heat to medium and simmer within 2-4 minutes. Stir occasionally, so it doesn't burn, then set aside.

4. Once the zoodles are finished, transfer it to a long piece of paper towel, cover with a different piece of paper towel, and then press out excess moisture.

5. Repeat the process with a fresh layer of paper towel over the top, then set aside. Beat the ricotta cheese, egg, and another pinch of pepper in a medium bowl, using a fork. Set aside.

6. For layer, spray the bottom of a slow cooker using cooking spray. Put in half of the turkey batter. Layer it with half the zucchini noodles in a single layer, then half the ricotta batter. Spread out the ricotta to "seal" in the zoodles.

7. Put half the cilantro on, then half the cabbage plus half the water chestnuts, finally, with half the mozzarella cheese.

8. Repeat the layers, except only use half of the rest of the mozzarella cheese on top. Then, add the diced red pepper on top of the last layer of mozzarella.

9. Cover your slow cooker and cook on low within 4-5 hours, or until everything is melted and the sides of the lasagna are brown. Sprinkle on the remaining cheese and let stand, covered until melted. Sprinkle with all the garnishes and devour!

Nutrition:

- Calories: 275
- Carbs: 13g
- Fat: 13g
- Protein: 26g

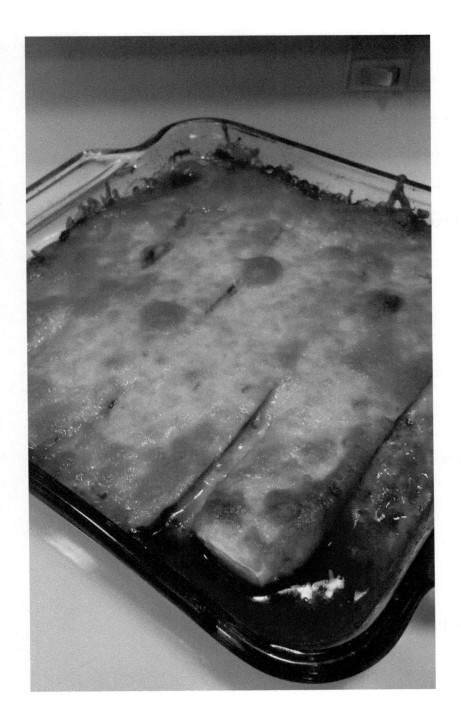

Keto Eggplants

Preparation Time: 15 minutes

Cooking Time: 7 hours

Servings: 14

Ingredients:

- 4 tbsps. olive oil
- 1 red onion
- 2 garlic cloves
- 1 lb. eggplant
- 7 ripe tomatoes
- 1 fennel bulb
- 4 sundried tomatoes
- 1 tsp. coriander seeds

Dressing:

- ¼ c. flat-leaf parsley
- ¼ c. basil
- 2 tsp. chives
- 2 tbsps. olive oil
- 1 juiced lemon

Topping:

- ½ c. toasted flaked almonds
- Keto bread for serving

Directions:

1. Peel the red onion and slice. Peel the garlic and crush it. Slice the bulb. Wash the tomatoes and cut. Wash parsley and chop, wash the basil leaves, chop the chives.

2. Squeeze the juice of a lemon. Open the crockpot, pour a little bit of olive oil into the crockpot, put the onions into the bottom, and add crushed garlic.

3. Slice the eggplant into thick slices and salt. Put them into the crockpot on top of the mix from onions and tomatoes, fennel, and sundried tomatoes.

4. Spread the coriander seeds, season well with salt and pepper. Cover and cook on low within 7 hours; the eggplant must be softened.

5. Prepare the dressing—mix parsley and basil, olive oil, juice of lemon, chives. Transfer the ready dish to a serving plate and drizzle with the dressing. Top with flaked almonds and serve with Keto bread.

Nutrition:

- Calories: 229
- Fat: 8.7g
- Protein: 31.7g
- Carbs: 4.7g

Italian Vegetable Bake

Preparation Time: 15 minutes

Cooking Time: 5 hours

Servings: 7

Ingredients:

- 3 garlic cloves
- 1 can tomato
- 1 bunch oregano
- ¼ tsp. chili flakes
- 11oz. baby aubergines
- 2 Courgettes
- ½ jar roasted red peppers
- 3 tomatoes
- 1 bunch basil
- Green salad

Directions:

1. Peel the garlic and mince. Chop tomatoes from the can. Wash the courgettes and slice, chop baby aubergines. Slice tomatoes. Open the crockpot, put the garlic, diced tomatoes, oregano leaves, chili, and some seasoning, add olive oil if necessary.

2. Add chopped aubergines, tomatoes, courgettes, red peppers, basil, and remaining oregano. Repeat vegetable layer, herb, and tomatoes. Push down well to compress, set on high for 5 hours. Serve with the basil leaves and the green salad.

Nutrition:
- Calories: 60
- Fat: 3.5g
- Protein: 2g
- Carbs: 6g

Spicy Maple Meatballs

Preparation Time: 15 minutes

Cooking Time: 5 hours

Servings: 11

Ingredients:

- 1 tbsp. olive oil
- ½ white onion
- 1 red bell pepper
- 1 green bell pepper
- 2 jalapeno peppers
- 1½ c. plain tomato sauce
- 1 c. maple syrup
- 2 tbsps. almond flour
- 2 tsp. ground allspice
- 1/8 tsp. liquid smoke
- 1 bag frozen vegan meatballs

Directions:

1. Peel the onion, chop it finely. Wash and slice peppers. Set aside. Add olive oil to the crockpot, add onion and peppers.

2. Take a medium bowl to add flour, maple syrup, tomato sauce, allspice, liquid smoke. Mix all until smooth consistency. Pour into the crockpot.

3. Add frozen meatballs. Cover and cook on low for 5 hours. The sauce should be thick and cover the meatballs. Serve warm over cauliflower rice.

Nutrition:
- Calories: 68
- Fat: 1.6g
- Protein: 7.2g
- Carbs: 6.6g

Spiced Cauliflower

Preparation Time: 10 minutes

Cooking Time: 2 hours

Servings: 13

Ingredients:

- 1 large cauliflower, cut into 1-inch pieces
- 1 medium onion, diced
- 1 medium tomato, dice
- 2 ginger roots, grate
- 2 garlic cloves
- 2 jalapeño peppers, sliced
- 1 tbsp cumin seeds
- ¼ tsp. cayenne pepper
- 1 tbsp. garam masala
- 1 tbsp. kosher salt
- 1 tsp. turmeric
- 3 tbsp. vegetable oil
- 1 tbsp. fresh cilantro, chop

Directions:

1. Put in the crockpot cauliflower florets, onion, tomato, ginger, garlic, peppers, masala, salt, turmeric, oil, and all the other fixing except fresh cilantro. Stir everything well. Cover and put on low for 2 hours. Serve with fresh cilantro.

Nutrition:

- Calories: 87
- Fat: 2.1g
- Protein: 10.3g
- Carbs: 7g

Garlic-Parmesan Asparagus

Preparation Time: 10 minutes

Cooking Time: 1 hour

Servings: 6

Ingredients:

- 2 tbsps. olive oil extra virgin
- 2 tsp. minced garlic
- 1 egg
- ½ tsp. garlic salt
- 12oz. fresh asparagus
- 1/3 cup of Parmesan cheese, shred
- pepper

Directions:

1. Take a medium-sized bowl combine oil, garlic, cracked egg, and salt. Whisk everything well. Cover the green beans and coat them well.

2. Spread the cooking spray over the crockpot's bottom, put the coated asparagus, season with the shredded cheese. Toss everything finely.

3. Cover and cook on high for 1 hour. Once the time is over, you may also season with the rest of the cheese.

Nutrition:

- Calories: 60
- Fat: 4.4g
- Protein: 2.2g
- Carbs: 4.7g

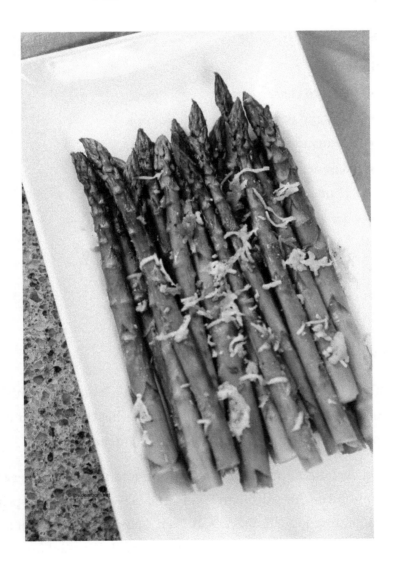

Spinach Artichoke Casserole

Preparation Time: 10 minutes

Cooking Time: 6 hours

Servings: 10

Ingredients:

- 8 large eggs
- 3/4 cup unsweetened almond milk
- 5 ounces fresh spinach chopped
- 6 ounces artichoke hearts chopped
- 1 cup grated parmesan
- 3 minced garlic cloves
- 1 tsp salt
- 1/2 tsp pepper
- 3/4 cup coconut flour
- 1 tbsp baking powder

Directions:

1. Oil the inside of a 6-quart slow cooker. In a large bowl, whisk the eggs, almond milk, spinach, artichoke hearts, 1/2 cup of the parmesan or nutritional yeast, garlic, salt, and pepper.

2. Add coconut flour and baking powder and whisk until very well combined. Spread mixture into the slow cooker and sprinkle remaining 1/2 cup parmesan over. Cook on high within 2 to 3 hours or low for 4 to 6 hours. Sprinkle with chopped fresh basil.

Nutrition:

- Calories: 141
- Fat: 7.1g
- Protein: 10g
- Carbs: 7.8g

French Onion Soup

Preparation Time: 10 minutes

Cooking Time: 4 hours

Servings: 8

Ingredients:

- 2 large white onions, sliced thin
- 6 cups low-sodium beef or bone broth
- 2 cups cheese, grated
- 1 tbsp ghee or butter
- 1 garlic clove, minced
- 1/2 tsp salt
- 1/2 tsp dried thyme
- 1/4 tsp pepper
- 1 bay leaf

Directions:

1. Add all the fixing except the cheese to the slow cooker. Stir to mix well. Cook high 3-4 hours, low 6-8. Remove bay leaf.

2. Preheat broiler. Ladle the soup evenly into bowls & top evenly with shredded cheese. Arrange bowls on a large baking sheet.

3. Place the baking sheet carefully under the broiler and broil a few minutes or until cheese is melted and slightly brown. Serve and enjoy!

Nutrition:

- Calories: 150
- Fat: 10.3g
- Protein: 10.4g
- Carbs: 4.2g

Vegan Rice and Beans

Preparation Time: 5 minutes

Cooking Time: 4 hours

Servings: 6

Ingredients:

- 2 packages frozen cauliflower rice (12oz each.)
- 2 cans black soybeans, drained
- 1/2 cup hulled hemp seeds
- 1 cup vegetable broth or stock
- 3 tbsp olive oil
- 2 tsp garlic powder
- 1 tsp onion powder
- 1 tsp cumin
- 1 tsp chili powder
- 1/2 tsp cayenne powder
- 1 tbsp Mexican oregano
- Garnishes of choice

Directions:

1. Add all the fixing except the Mexican oregano to the slow cooker, then mix around as best as possible. Let cook on High within 3-4 hours, until the "rice" is tender. Stir in oregano, then serve.

Nutrition:

- Calories: 299
- Fat: 20.2g
- Protein: 19.3g
- Carbs: 4.9g

Broccoli Parmesan Soup

Preparation Time: 10 minutes

Cooking Time: 2 hours

Servings: 12

Ingredients:

- 2 cups of water
- 2 cups of chicken broth
- 5 cups of fresh broccoli florets, chopped
- 8oz. softened cream cheese
- 1 cup whipping cream
- 1/2 cup Parmesan cheese
- 2 ½ cups shredded Cheddar cheese
- 2 tbsp of softened unsalted butter
- Dash of thyme
- Salt and pepper to taste

Directions:

1. In your slow cooker, put the butter, softened cream cheese, whipping cream, chicken broth, water, and mix well. Once thoroughly combined, add the parmesan cheese.

2. Put the chopped broccoli crowns, thyme. Cover and cook on low within 3 hours or medium-high for 80 minutes.

3. Then simply give the soup a good stir and then add the 2 1/2 cups of shredded cheddar cheese. Stir a few times, allowing the

cheddar cheese to melt completely. Add the salt and pepper to taste.

Nutrition:

- Calories: 230
- Fat: 20g
- Protein: 9.8g
- Carbs: 3.8g

Zucchini Pasta

Preparation time: 15 minutes

Cooking time: 1 hour

Servings: 4

Ingredients:

- 2 zucchinis
- 1 teaspoon dried oregano
- 1 teaspoon dried basil
- 2 tablespoons butter
- ¼ teaspoon salt
- 5 tablespoons water

Directions:

1. Peel the zucchini and spiralize it with a veggie spiralizer. Dissolve the butter and mix it with the dried oregano, dried basil, salt, and water.

2. Place the spiralized zucchini in the slow cooker and add the spice mixture. Close the lid and cook the meal for 1 hour on low. Let the cooked pasta cool slightly. Serve it!

Nutrition:

- Calories: 68
- Fat: 6g
- Carbs: 3.5g
- Protein: 1.3g

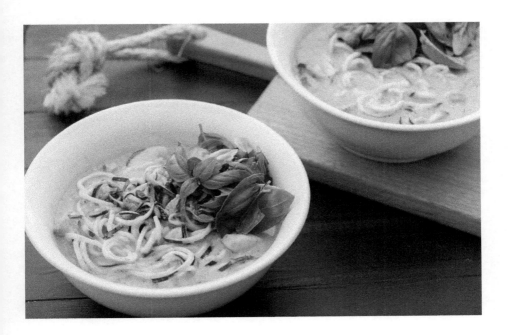

Lightning Source UK Ltd.
Milton Keynes UK
UKHW020817170621
385664UK00001B/86